Plant-Based Diet

The Plant-Based Diet for Beginners_ What Is a Plant-Based Diet_ Plant-Based Diet vs. Vegan, Plant-Based Diet Benefits, and Plant-Based Diet Recipes

By

Michael J. York

The information provided herein is stated to be truthful and consistent, in that any liability, in terms of inattention or otherwise, by any usage or abuse of any policies, processes, or directions contained within is the solitary and utter responsibility of the recipient reader. Under no circumstances will any legal responsibility or blame be held against the publisher for any reparation, damages, or monetary loss due to the information herein, either directly or indirectly.

Respective authors own all copyrights not held by the publisher.

The information herein is offered for informational purposes solely, and is universal as so. The presentation of the information is without contract or any type of guarantee assurance.

The trademarks that are used are without any consent, and the publication of the trademark is without permission or backing by the trademark owner. All trademarks and brands within this book are for clarifying purposes only and are the owned by the owners themselves, not affiliated with this document.

Table of contents

Introduction

It is only until recently that more and more people are starting to embrace the plant-based diet lifestyle. As to what exactly has drawn tens of millions of people into this lifestyle is debatable. However, there is growing evidence demonstrating that following a primarily plant-based diet lifestyle leads to better weight control and general health, free of many chronic diseases. This book will take you through the basics of this lifestyle, its benefits and why it works, as well as give ideas on how you can revamp your pantry and start whipping up delectable plant-based dishes. Whether you are new to this lifestyle or familiar with it, this book is definitely a treasure. Enjoy!

Chapter 1: The Basics of a Plant-Based Diet

1.1 What Is A Plant-Based Diet?

A lot of people are doing it; a lot of people are talking about it, but there is still a lot of confusion about what a whole food plant-based diet really means. Because we break food into its macronutrients: carbohydrates, proteins, and fats; most of us get confused about how to eat. What if we could put back together those macronutrients again so that you can free your mind of confusion and stress?

Simplicity is the key here.

Whole foods are unprocessed foods that come from the earth. Now, we do eat some minimally processed foods on a whole foods plant-based diet such as whole bread, whole wheat pasta, tofu, non-dairy milk and some nuts and seed butter. All these are fine as long as they are minimally processed. So, here are the different categories: Whole grains Legumes   (basically lentils and beans)

Fruits and vegetables   Nuts and seeds (including nut butter)   Herbs and spices All the above-mentioned categories make up a whole foods plant-based diet. Where the fun comes in is in how you prepare them; how you season and cook them; and how you mix and match to give them great flavor and variety in your meals. There are chapters in this book dedicated to plant-based recipes which can give you an idea of what you can whip up real quick in your kitchen or those special meals you can prepare for the family. As long as you are eating foods like these on a regular basis, you can forget about carbs, protein and fat forever.

Now, some people might say, "well, I can't eat soy" or "I don't like tofu" and so on. Well, the beauty of a whole food plant based diet is that if you don't like a certain food, like in this case, soy, then you don't have to consume it. It is not a necessary component in a whole food plant-based diet. You can have brown rice

instead of oats, quinoa instead of wheat; I'm sure you catch the drift now. It doesn't really matter. Just find something that suits you.

Just because you have made the decision to adopt a plant-based diet lifestyle, doesn't mean that is a healthy diet. Plant-based diets have their fair share of junk and other unhealthy eats; case and point, regular consumption of veggie pizzas and non-dairy ice cream. Staying healthy requires you to eat healthy foods – even within a plant-based diet setting.

1.2 Why You Need to Cut Back On Processed and Animal-Based Products

You've probably heard time and time again that processed food is bad for you. "Avoid preservatives; avoid processed foods"; however, no one ever really gives you any real or solid information on why you should avoid them and why they are dangerous. So let's break it down so that you can fully understand why you should avoid these culprits.

They have huge addictive properties

As humans, we really have a strong tendency to be addicted to certain foods, but the fact is that it's not entirely our fault.

Practically all of the unhealthy eats we indulge in, from time to time, activate our brains dopamine neurotransmitter. This makes the brain feel "good" but only for a short period of time. This also creates an addiction tendency; that is why someone will always find themselves going back for another candy bar – even though they don't really need it. You can avoid all this by removing that stimulus altogether.

They are loaded sugar and high fructose corn syrup

Processed and animal-based products are loaded with sugars and high fructose corn syrup which have close to zero nutritional value. More and more studies are now proving what a lot of people suspected all along; that genetically modified foods cause gut inflammation which in turn makes it harder for the body to absorb essential nutrients. The downside of your body failing to properly absorb essential nutrients, from muscle loss and brain fog to fat gain, cannot be stressed enough.

They are loaded with refined carbohydrates

Processed foods and animal-based products are loaded with refined carbs. Yes, it is a fact that your body needs carbs to provide energy to run body functions.

However, refining carbs eliminates the essential nutrients; in the way that refining whole grains eliminates the whole grain component. What you are left with after refining is what's referred to as "empty" carbs. These can have a negative impact on your metabolism by spiking your blood sugar and insulin levels.

They are loaded with artificial ingredients

When your body is consuming artificial ingredients, it treats them as a foreign object. They essentially become an invader. Your body isn't used to recognizing things like sucralose or these artificial sweeteners. So, your body does what it does best. It triggers an immune response which lowers your resistance making you vulnerable to diseases. The focus and energy spent by your body in protecting your immune system could otherwise be diverted elsewhere.

They contain components that cause a hyper reward sense in your body

What this means is that they contain components like monosodium glutamate (MSG), components of high fructose corn syrup and certain dyes that can actually carve addictive properties. They stimulate your body to get a reward out of it. MSG, for instance, is in a lot of pre-packaged pastries. What this does is that it stimulates your taste buds to enjoy the taste. It becomes psychological just by the way your brain communicates with your taste buds.

This reward-based system makes your body want more and more of it putting

you at a serious risk of caloric overconsumption.

What about animal protein? Often times the term "low quality" is thrown around to refer to plant proteins since they tend to have lower amounts of essential amino acids compared to animal protein. What most people do not realize is that more essential amino acids can be quite damaging to your health. So, let's quickly explain how.

Animal Protein Lacks Fiber

In their quest to load up on more animal protein most people end up displacing the plant protein that they already had. This is bad because unlike plant protein, animal protein often lacks in fiber, antioxidants, and phytonutrients. Fiber deficiency is quite common across different communities and societies in the world. In the USA, for instance, according to the Institute of Medicine, the average adult consumes just about 15 grams of fiber per day against the recommended 38 grams. Lack of adequate dietary fiber intake is associated with an increased risk of colon and breast cancers, as well as Crohn's disease, heart disease, and constipation.

Animal protein causes a spike in IGF-1

IGF-1 is the hormone insulin-like growth factor-1. It stimulates cell division and growth, which may sound like a good thing but it also stimulates the growth of cancer cells. Higher blood levels of IGF-1 are thus associated with increased cancer risks, malignancy, and proliferation.

Animal Protein causes an increase in Phosphorus

Animal protein contains high levels of phosphorus. Our bodies normalize the high levels of phosphorus by secreting a hormone called fibroblast growth factor 23 (FGF23). This hormone has been found to be harmful to our blood vessels,

thanks to a 2013 study titled, "Circulating Fibroblast Growth Factor 23 Is Associated with Angiographic Severity and Extent of Coronary Artery Disease". FGF23 has also been found to cause irregular enlargement of cardiac muscles – a risk factor for heart failure and even death in extreme cases.

Given all the issues, the "high quality" aspect of animal protein might be more appropriately described as "high risk" instead. Unlike caffeine, which you will experience withdrawal once you cut it off completely, processed foods can be cut off instantaneously. Perhaps the one thing that you'll miss is the convenience of not having to prepare every meal from scratch.

1.3 Plant-Based Diet vs. Vegan

It is quite common for people to mistake a vegan diet for a plant-based diet or vice versa. Well, even though both diets share similarities, they are not exactly the same. So let's break it down real quick.

Vegan

A vegan diet is one that contains no animal-based products. This includes meat, dairy, eggs as well as animal-derived products or ingredients such as honey.

Someone who describes themselves as a vegan carries over this perspective into their everyday life. What this means is that they do not use or promote the use of clothes, shoes, accessories, shampoo, and makeups that have been made using material that comes from animals. Examples here include wool, beeswax, leather, gelatin, silk, and lanolin.

The motivation for people to lead a veganism lifestyle often stems from a desire to make a stand and fight against animal mistreatment and poor ethical treatment of animals as well as to promote animal rights.

Plant Based Diet

A whole food plant based diet in the other hand shares a similarity with veganism in the sense that it also does not promote dietary consumption of animal-based products. This includes dairy, meat, and eggs. What's more is that, unlike the vegan diet, processed foods, white flour, oils and refined sugars are not part of the diet. The idea here is to make a diet out of minimally processed to unprocessed fruits, veggies, whole grains, nuts, seeds, and legumes. So, there will be NO Oreo cookies for you.

Whole-food plant-based diet followers are often driven by the health benefits it brings. It is a diet that has very little to do with restricting calories or counting

macros but mostly to do with preventing and reversing illnesses.

1.4 Getting Started on a Whole Food Plant-Based Diet

A common misconception among many people – even some of those in the health and fitness industry is that anyone who switches to a plant-based diet automatically becomes super healthy. There are tons of plant-based junk foods out there such as non-dairy ice cream and frozen veggie pizza, which can really derail your health goals if you are constantly consuming them. Committing to healthy foods is the only way that you can achieve health benefits. On the other hand, these plant-based snacks do play a role in keeping you motivated. They should be consumed in moderation, sparingly and in small bits. As you will come to see later on in this book, there is a chapter dedicated to giving ideas on plant-based snacks you can whip up at home. So, without further ado, this is how you get started on a whole food plant-based recipe.

Decide What a Plant-Based Diet Means for You Making a decision to structure how your plant-based diet is going to look is the first step, and it is going to help you transition from your current diet outlook. This is something that is really personal and varies from one person to the other. While some people decide that they will not tolerate any animal products at all, some make do with tiny bits of dairy or meat occasionally. It is really up to you to decide what and how you want your plant-based diet to look like. The most important thing is that whole plant-based foods have to make a great majority of your diet.

Understand What You Are Eating All right, now that you've gotten the decision part down, your next task is going to involve a lot of analysis on your part. What do we mean by this? Well, if this is your first time trying out the plant-based diet, you may be surprised by the number of foods, especially packaged foods, which contain animal products. You will find yourself nurturing the habit of reading labels while you are shopping. Turns out, lots of pre- packaged foods have animal products in them, so if you want to stick only to plant products for your new diet, you'll need to keep a keen eye on ingredient labels. Perhaps you decided to allow some amount of animal products in your diet; well, you are still going to have to watch out for foods loaded with fats, sugars, sodium, preservatives and other things that could potentially impact your healthy diet.

Find Revamped Versions of Your Favorite Recipes I'm sure you have a number of favorite dishes that are not necessarily plant-based. For most people, leaving all that behind is usually the hardest part. However, there is still a way you could meet halfway. Take some time to ponder what you like about those non-plant based meals. Think along the lines of flavor, texture, versatility and so on; and look for swaps in the whole food plant-based diet that can fulfill what you will be missing. Just to give you some insight into what I mean, here are a couple of examples:

Crumbled or blended tofu would make for a decent filling in both sweet and savory dishes just like ricotta cheese would in lasagna.

Lentils go particularly well with saucy dishes that are typically associated with meatloaf and Bolognese.

As you read on, you will come across a chapter dedicated to an assortment of delectable main course recipes that are purely plant-based. All in all, when this is executed right, you will not even miss your non-plant based favorite meals.

Build a Support Network

Building any new habit is tough, but it doesn't have to be. Find yourself some friends, or even relatives, who are willing to lead this lifestyle with you. This will help you stay focused and motivated while also providing emotional support and some form of accountability. You can do fun stuff like trying out and sharing new recipes with these friends or even hitting up restaurants that offer a variety of plant-based options. You can even go a step further and look up local plant- based groups on social media to help you expand your knowledge and support network.

Chapter 2: What You Stand to Gain from a Plant- Based Diet

2.1 The Benefits of Going Plant-Based

More and more people are becoming aware of the ability of a whole food plant based diet to help alleviate and even cure many chronic diseases such as heart disease, type 2 diabetes, arthritis, cancers, autoimmune disease, kidney stones, inflammatory bowel diseases and many more. Not to mention, a plant-based diet is more economical – especially when you buy local organic produce that is in season. So let's check out some of the benefits of going plant-based.

It Lowers Blood Pressure

Plant-based foods tend to have a higher amount of potassium whose benefits, notably include: reducing blood pressure and alleviating stress and anxiety. Some foods rich in potassium include legumes, nuts, seeds, whole grains, and fruits. Meat, on the other hand, contains very little to no potassium.

It Lowers Cholesterol

Plants contain NO cholesterol – even the saturated sources like cacao and coconut.

Leading a plant-based lifestyle will, therefore, help you lower the levels of cholesterol in your body leading to reduced risks of heart disease.

Checks Your Blood Sugar Levels

Plant-based foods tend to have a lot of fiber. This helps slow down the absorption of sugars into the bloodstream as well as keep you feeling full for longer periods of time. It also helps balance out your blood cortisol levels thereby reducing stress.

It Helps Prevent and Fight Off Chronic Diseases

In societies where a majority of people lead a plant-based lifestyle the rates of chronic diseases such as cancer, obesity, and diabetes are usually very low. This diet has also been proven to lengthen the lives of those already suffering from these chronic diseases.

It Is Good for Weight Loss

Consuming whole plant-based foods make it easier to cut off excess weight and maintain a healthier weight without having to involve calorie restrictions. This is because Weight loss naturally occurs when you consume more fiber, vitamins, and minerals than you do animal fats and proteins.

2.2 What Some Influential People Think of a Plant-Based Lifestyle

Whether we like to admit it or not, celebrities do have a lot of fame and power, which can either be used to promote good or promote evil. Going plant-based can be quite a daunting experience as it often comes with a health and lifestyle overhaul, however, nowadays it's become an increasingly popular diet – and a host of stars have made the change. We have already explored some of the numerous benefits of going plant-based. Some celebrities are passively plant- based diet followers; this means that they are not celebrities because of their diet views, but became a celebrity as a result of something else like their music or roles in the film industry. Others are active plant-based diet followers whose claim to fame is adding something of value to the conversation of a plant-based diet and lifestyle. Let's look at some celebrities who subscribe to this lifestyle and what they have to say.

Liam Hemsworth who's an acclaimed actor known for many film roles among which include, The Hunger Games once said this to Men's Fitness Magazine about the plant-based diet, "I feel nothing but positive, mentally and physically. I love it. I feel like it also has a kind of a domino effect on the rest of my life".

Jennifer Lopez, a well-known and talented singer and actress, after the giving birth to her twins, had this to say about plant-based diet: "It is a real change, but more than that I feel better and people are like 'Your energy's better'."

Jenna Dewan Tatum made the jump from vegetarian to vegan a couple of years ago. She says, "After going vegan, I felt so much better. My skin cleared up, I had a ton more energy and I just felt clearer in the head".

Ariana Grande is yet another plant-based diet follower who shares a trick she employs when dining out. She says, "It is tricky dining out, but I just stick to what I know – veggies, fruit and salad - then when I get home I'll have

something else."

Taj McWilliams-Franklin, a professional basketball player, was quoted in a 2008 interview about why she decided to go plant-based saying, "I just wanted to make sure I had a healthy body because I wanted to continue playing for a longer period than most of my peers."

2.3 What to Look Out For When Adopting this Lifestyle

For most people looking to go plant-based, protein is always a major concern. There is this notion that's perpetuated by the mainstream media backed by big meat producers that protein is only found in meat. Well, that's just not true.

Traditional staples such as nuts, beans, oats and brown rice come with a lot of protein.

Often times, nutrients like calcium are also marketed as coming from only animal-based sources. The truth is that foods like kale, broccoli, and almonds contain lots of calcium. Ask yourself this, if calcium comes from meat, then where did the animal get it from? It's definitely from the greens they eat.

The major concern for most plant-based diet followers is usually vitamin B12. B12, for everyone, is usually found in fortified products, especially cereals and plant-based milk. However, those shouldn't be relied on to get enough of this important vitamin. The best option is to take a liquid or sublingual vitamin B12 supplement simply; just to make sure that there are no issues.

You can adopt a healthy plant-based lifestyle by basing your diet around cooked and raw foods filled with leafy and colorful veggies. These will provide your body with the minerals, vitamins, and antioxidants it needs.

Chapter 3: Planning and Stocking Your Pantry

3.1 A Quick word on Pantry Planning

As you transition into a whole-food, plant-based lifestyle, you don't have to worry about stocking. Your local farmer's market or grocery store should provide you with everything you need. Consider getting sets of transparent jars which you will use to store your food. This will make for a presentable look in your pantry. Typically, you will have some shelves dedicated to storage of grains, nuts, beans, spices, herbs and so on.

3.2 Stock Your Pantry: Food Guide for a Plant-Based Diet

Foods to Stock Non-Starchy Vegetables

Leafy greens (Kale, Spinach, Butter Lettuce etc.) Broccoli

Zucchini Eggplant Tomatoes

Starchy Vegetables

All kinds of potatoes Whole corn

Legumes (all beans and lentils) Root vegetables

Quinoa

Fruits

All whole fruits (avoid dried and juiced fruits)

Whole Grains

100% whole wheat, brown rice, and oats

Beverages

Water Green tea

Unsweetened plant-based milk Decaffeinated coffee and tea

Spices

All spices

Omega 3 Sources

Ground flax seed Chia seeds

Nuts

Peanuts Almonds Cashews Walnuts

Foods to Consume Sparingly

Avocadoes Coconuts Sesame seeds Sunflower seeds Pumpkin seeds Dried fruit

Added sweeteners (maple syrup, fruit juice concentrate, and natural sugars)

Caffeinated tea and coffee Alcoholic beverages

Refined soy protein and wheat protein

Foods to Avoid Meat

Fish Poultry Seafood Red meat

Processed meat

Dairy

Yogurt Milk Cheese Cream

Half and half Buttermilk

Added Fats

Liquid oils Coconut oil Margarine Butter

Beverages

Soda Fruit juice

Sports drinks Energy drinks

Blended coffee and tea drinks

Refined Flours

All wheat flours that are not 100% whole wheat

Vegan Replacement Foods

Vegan "cheese" or vegan "meats" containing any oil

Miscellaneous

Eggs Candy bars Pastries Cookies Cakes Energy bars

3.3 A Quick Word on Labels

When shopping to restock your pantry, always keep in mind that the goal is not to eat a lot of foods that require packaging or labels. However, it is normal to have that packaged food item on your list occasionally. When this does happen, these tips will help you stay vigilant and ensure a healthy shopping experience.

Do Not Believe Company Claims Terms like 'low in fat' or '50% less sodium' are very popular on packaged foods. They don't really mean anything. What you should instead be focusing on is the ingredient list and the nutrition label. Just because a bag of potato chips has been labeled as having 40% less sodium doesn't mean that it is healthy.

It could very well be still high in sodium or come with a host of other unwanted ingredients. The same goes for products labeled as "low-fat."

Make a Habit of Checking the Ingredient List As a general rule, the fewer ingredients there are, the healthier the food is. Such foods often have very few to no additives and preservatives which is good for your health. When you see the ingredients list containing a lot of words ending in "-ose," this is often an indicator that the food contains a lot of sugar. Also, check if there are any animal products on the ingredient list.

Chapter 4: Breakfast and Brunch Recipes

Maple Granola with Banana Whipped Topping

Ingredients

2 cups of rolled oats

¼ cup of raw sunflower seeds

¼ cup of raw pumpkin seeds

¼ cup of raw unsweetened shredded dried coconut

¼ cup chopped walnuts

¼ cup raw or toasted wheat germ 1 teaspoon ground cinnamon

½ cup maple syrup

¾ cup raisins

Banana Whipped Topping, optional For Banana Whipped Topping

8 ounces soft or firm regular tofu, drained (sprouted variety is preferred)

1   ripe banana

2   tablespoons maple syrup, plus more as needed

Instructions

i.   Line a baking sheet with parchment paper and preheat your oven to 330 degrees F.

ii.   Combine oats, pumpkin seeds, walnuts, sunflower seeds, cinnamon and wheat germ in a bowl along with maple syrup.

iii.   Now in your baking sheet, spread the mixture evenly and bake for about 20 minutes.

iv.   Stir in raisins and bake for another 5 minutes until the oats are

golden.

v.   Transfer to another baking sheet or tray and let it cool. You can serve it with banana toppings.

For Topping

Combine topping ingredients in a blender until smooth. Add maple syrup as desired.

Chickpea Flour Scramble Ingredients Chickpea flour batter:

½ cup of chickpea flour or use ½ cup + 1 or 2 tablespoons of more gram flour

½ cup of water

1 tablespoon of nutritional yeast 1 tablespoon of flaxseed meal

½ teaspoon of baking powder

¼ teaspoon of salt

¼ teaspoon of turmeric

¼ teaspoon or less paprika

1/8 teaspoon of Indian Sulphur black salt for the eggy flavor Generous dash of black pepper

For Veggies:

1   teaspoon of oil divided 1 clove of garlic

¼ cup chopped onions

2   tablespoons each of asparagus green bell pepper, zucchini or other veggies.

½ green chili, chopped

2 tablespoons of chopped red bell pepper or tomato Cilantro and black pepper for garnish

Instructions

i.   Blend all the ingredients under chickpea flour batter and keep aside. You can also use lentil batter from my lentil frittata.

ii.   Heat ½ teaspoon of oil in a skillet over medium heat. Add onion and garlic and cook for about 3 minutes until translucent.

iii.   Add veggies, chili and cook for another 2 mins, then add spices and greens.

iv.   Cover the veggies with the chickpea flour batter and continue cooking while adding olive oil.

v.   Since the mixture tends to get doughy, be sure to scrap the bottom. Cook until the edges dry out. This should take about 5 minutes.

vi.   Turn off the stove and break the food into smaller chunks then season with salt and pepper. You can garnish with cilantro if you like. Serve with toast or tacos.

Peanut Butter and Jam Porridge Ingredients Peanut butter granola

½ cup of rolled oats or an assortment of cereals/nuts/seeds in your pantry

1 tablespoon peanut butter

1 teaspoon of rice malt syrup

Raspberry chia jam

¼ cup raspberries

1 tablespoon chia seeds

Porridge

⅔ Cup of rolled oats 1½ cup of coconut milk

2 tablespoon of peanut butter (optional) 1 banana, mashed (optional)

Other toppings

2 tablespoon of peanut butter

Whatever you desire! (Such as cacao nibs, coconut syrup, coconut and frozen berries)

Instructions

i.   Preheat oven to 360°F.

ii.   Combine granola ingredients in a baking sheet and bake for about 10 minutes (or until golden brown)

iii.   Mash raspberries and mix in chia seeds then set it aside.

iv.   Combine all porridge ingredients in a saucepan and bring to boil. Stir occasionally to maintain its smoothness.

v.   Separate the porridge into 2 bowls and add granola, chia seeds, and peanut butter as desired.

Banana Almond Granola Ingredients

8 cups rolled oats

2 cups pitted and chopped dates

2 ripe bananas, peeled and chopped 1 teaspoon almond extract

1 teaspoon salt

1   cup slivered almonds, toasted (optional)

Instructions

i.   Preheat the oven to 275°F.

ii.   Line a baking sheet with parchment paper.

iii.   Cook dates covered with water in a saucepan over medium heat for about 10 minutes. Make sure the dates do not stick on the pan.

iv.   Take the mixture off heat and in a blender, combine it with almond extract, bananas and salt until creamy.

v.   Add oats to the date mixture and spread out on the baking sheet. Bake for about 45 minutes – occasionally stirring.

vi.   Remove from oven and let it cool. Enjoy.

Polenta with Pears and Cranberries Ingredients

¼ cup of brown rice syrup

2   pears, peeled, cored, and diced 1 cup of fresh or dried cranberries 1 teaspoon ground cinnamon

1   batch Basic Polenta, kept warm

Instructions

i.   In a medium saucepan, combine the brown rice syrup, cranberries, pears and cinnamon. Cook until the pears are tender.

ii.   Divide as desired and top with pear compote.

Fruit and Nut Oatmeal Ingredients

¾ cup of rolled oats

¼ teaspoon ground cinnamon Pinch of sea salt

¼ cup fresh berries (optional)

½ ripe banana, sliced (optional)

2   tablespoons of chopped nuts, such as walnuts, pecans, or cashews (optional)

2 tablespoons of dried fruit, such as raisins, cranberries, chopped apples, chopped

Apricots (optional) Maple syrup (optional)

Instructions

i.   Cook oats in water in a saucepan until it starts boiling. Reduce the heat and let it simmer for about 5 minutes.

ii.   Add cinnamon and salt – stirring. Top with berries and fruits and serve while hot.

Red Pesto and Kale Porridge Ingredients

½ cup of oats

½ cup of couscous

2 cups of veggie stock (or water) 1 teaspoon of dried oregano

1 teaspoon of dried basil 1 cup of chopped kale

1 cup of sliced cherry tomatoes 1 scallion

1 teaspoon of tahini

1 tablespoon of pesto of your choice 2 tablespoons of nutritional yeast

1   tablespoon of pumpkin seed 1 tablespoon of hemp seed Salt and pepper to taste

Instructions

i.   Cook oats, couscous, vegetable stock, oregano, basil, salt and pepper in a small pot on medium heat for about 5 minutes stirring occasionally.

ii.   Once it becomes creamy, add scallions, chopped kale, and tomatoes. Stir in pesto, yeast, and tahini.

iii.   Top with some cherry tomatoes hemp seeds and pumpkin and serve it warm.

Spicy Tofu Scramble Ingredients

350g of firm tofu

2   small spring onions, sliced

1 large garlic clove, finely chopped 10 cherry tomatoes, halved

½ fresh red chili, sliced 1 avocado, sliced

1 teaspoon of ground turmeric 2 teaspoon of ground black salt Salt & pepper to taste

1 to 2 tablespoons of olive oil

8 slices of gluten-free bread, toasted

Instructions

i.   Sauté garlic in olive oil in a pan.

ii.   Add in tomatoes and cook until they're soft then remove the mixture from the pan.

iii.   Under a grill, toast bread slices. Sauté some onions and chili seeds on low-medium heat until they soften and add tofu.

iv.   Sprinkle with turmeric and black salt and stir it for a couple of minutes. Finally, add tomatoes and garlic back to the pan to warm up.

v.   Add the tofu scramble onto the toasted bread slices and decorate with avocado. Season as desired. Enjoy!

Green Chia Pudding Ingredients

1 Medjool date with pit removed

1 cup non-dairy milk organic soy, almond, or coconut 1 handful fresh spinach

3 tablespoons of chia seeds

Fruit for topping banana, kiwi, mango or berries

Instructions

i.   Combine the dates, milk, and spinach in a blender until smooth then add it to chia seeds in a medium bowl.

ii.   Store in the refrigerator for up to overnight.

iii.   Top with fruit before serving.

Turmeric Steel Cut Oats Ingredients

¼ teaspoon of olive oil

½ cup of steel cut oats use certified gluten-free if needed 1½ cup of water 2 cups for a thinner consistency

1   cup of non-dairy milk 1/3 teaspoon of turmeric

½ teaspoon of cinnamon

¼ teaspoon of cardamom Salt to taste

2   tablespoons or more, of maple or other sweetener of your choice

Instructions

i.   Toast oats in oil in a saucepan for a couple of minutes.

ii.   Add water and milk and bring it to a boil before letting it simmer.

iii.   Mix in the spices, salt, and maple and cook for about 8 minutes or until the oats are cooked to preference.

iv.   Taste and adjust sweet, and flavors as desired then let it cool to thicken. You can serve warm or chilled.

v.   Garnish with strawberries, dried fruit or chia seeds.

Conclusion

I believe now you understand how a plant-based diet lifestyle can be beneficial to you. I hope that the book answered all questions you may have heard about this style of dieting and that you can start to make it work for you. If you are still hesitant about entirely giving up animal products, you don't have to. The main take away here is that you make plant-based meals the main part of your diet as you make baby steps to transition into a full plant-based lifestyle. You will soon realize that your body and mind start to feel better, stronger and healthier. You can't fix your health until you fix your diet!

If you enjoyed learning about the plant-based diet, I would be forever grateful if you could leave a review on Amazon. Reviews are the best way to help your fellow readers find the good books so make sure to help them out!